Yoga for the Brain

Increase Your Brain Power with Yoga and Slow Down Brain Aging with Super Brain Yoga

Noah Miller

Contents

Introduction

Thank you for downloading *Yoga for the Brain*. This book offers readers a natural solution to a major health condition that is alarmingly on the rise at present: brain aging.

While it is true that the brain ages as a person ages, it doesn't happen at the same rate for everyone. Brain shrinkage is a natural process, but not everyone suffers negative consequences. Still, studies prove that disorders associated with brain aging are more common now than in the past. You will discover some of the best yoga for a healthy life and quality aging. Needless to say, exercise plays a vital role in keeping yourself healthy. And when it comes to exercise, what could be better than this ancient art that has been practiced for thousands of years?

In this book, discover:

- Factors influencing brain aging
- How yoga boosts brain power
- The best yoga poses for boosting brain health and how to perform them, with detailed instructions, benefits, and images
- The best breathing techniques for brain health and meditation
- One particular ancient practice that was once a daily routine in the land of yoga—and its immense benefits: super brain yoga.

I sincerely hope this guide will help seniors of today and tomorrow live life to the fullest with optimum quality.

Let's get started!

Brain and Aging

Why do we feel amazed when we meet a senior citizen with astounding memory power? It is popularly believed that brain function declines as one ages and hence memory power is compromised in seniors. But while it is true that a section of the older generation has issues related to memory, a sizable majority of older people possess perfectly sound memory power. Hence, it is clear that brain aging does not affect all older people uniformly. Some of the factors that play a role in healthy brain aging include regular exercise, diet and a healthy lifestyle.

The Aging of the Brain

The process of aging causes a number of changes in your physical and mental makeup, and the brain is no exception to the impact of aging. Aging causes structural, functional and biochemical changes in the brain.

The major structural changes in the brain as one ages include shrinkage, particularly of the prefrontal cortex, and thinning of cortical density, which affect memory and cognitive function. Loss of brain plasticity, that is, the brain's ability to modify its structure and function, is also seen.

Brain aging involves biochemical changes as well. Lower levels of dopamine may result in increased rigidity, which is why lower flexibility levels are common in seniors. Low serotonin levels, a contributor to depression, are also associated with brain aging.

Cerebral blood flow decreases with age, causing mental decline. White matter lesions that show up in seniors may influence both physical and mental performance. However, white matter lesions are also seen in seniors with sound cognitive health. These lesions are also linked with health conditions including cardiovascular disease.

Changes in neural network stimulation are observed in the elderly. The change in the pattern of stimulation means that seniors must summon up increased brain activity to perform any cognitive function.

The length of myelinated axons greatly decreases as the brain ages, leading to neurological conditions. Glucose metabolism may also be affected. Glucose metabolism is vital for brain function, and hence its disruption may lead to brain disorders.

Complications Associated With Brain Aging

One of the most commonly known conditions associated with aging is reduced memory power. The ability to remember names or recall a past event or date is compromised in a good number of seniors. It also becomes harder to maintain focus. Depression is yet another common symptom found in seniors, although it is not an inevitable part of growing old. Depression can be caused by certain health conditions or environmental factors. Elderly people with sound health and leading contended lives are usually free from depression.

Apart from these common conditions, there are certain more severe complications that can greatly affect the quality of life of seniors.

Dementia
Dementia is one of the most common brain disorders associated with aging. Dementia impairs the ability to communicate, recall and rationalize. Mental ability declines to an extent that it interferes with routine activities.

Alzheimer's Disease
Alzheimer's disease is the most common form of dementia. Alzheimer's can drastically affect quality of life. Victims may forget how to perform basic tasks such as brushing the teeth and combing the hair. Those with Alzheimer's tend to get lost when away from home on their own, as they lose their ability to remember places. Taking care of a person with Alzheimer's also poses a tough challenge, as the caregiver becomes a helpless witness as the condition deprives the person of certain aspects of her personality.

Parkinson's Disease

In the advanced stage, Parkinson's can cause dementia. Well before that, it deteriorates motor function, which causes tremors, gradually leads to compromised movements, and eventually confines the person to a wheelchair. Sleep pattern disorders and depression are some of the other symptoms. Although Parkinson's is not fatal, the complications can be very severe.

Stroke

Stroke occurs when blood flow to the brain is interrupted. It can occur in any part of the brain. The effects depend on the part of the brain affected and the intensity of the stroke. Stroke in the right brain paralyses the left side of the body and affects vision, while stroke in the left brain paralyses the right side of the body and affects speech. Stroke in the brainstem can affect the entire body below the neck.

While seniors are susceptible to the conditions mentioned above, a healthy lifestyle helps preserve quality of life as one ages. For those with the right attitude towards life, age is nothing but a number.

Factors Influencing Aging of Brain

Various factors play a role in how the brain ages. Strokes, Parkinson's, dementia and the like were not as common in the past as they are now, which highlights the fact that lifestyle has a role in how your brain ages. Factors which influence brain aging include:

Genetics

The risk of experiencing a health condition is higher if it runs in the family. Stroke, dementia, Parkinson's and Alzheimer's can be hereditary. According to studies, the onset of Alzheimer's in a son or daughter is impacted by when a parent began experiencing the symptoms of the condition.

Sedentary Lifestyle

A life devoid of exercise is a life of compromised cognitive function in the later stages. Sedentary behavior shrinks the brain, thus contributing to cognitive decline. The impact is worse when a person is at high risk of heart conditions, as being sedentary in such cases can speed up brain aging.

Diet

A healthy diet goes a long way in preserving brain health. A diet rich in omega-3 fatty acids supports cognitive function. The right type of diet, in combination with regular exercise, helps to maintain cognitive health as one ages. Getting enough of the right nutrients on a regular basis improves memory power and prevents cognitive decline.

Exercise, In All Forms Possible

Exercise helps to maintain brain health by stimulating brain chemicals and promoting blood flow to the brain. Regular exercise also helps to maintain greater brain volume, which otherwise shrinks during old age, causing lower cognitive performance.

Yoga is considered one of the best forms of exercise for promoting optimal health, both physical and mental. Brain exercises have been proven to prevent or postpone dementia and other neurodegenerative disorders. Exercise thus plays an influential role in preventing brain aging.

Can Yoga Reverse Brain Aging?

Yoga, the ancient art practiced around the world, evolved thousands of years ago. Yoga is practiced to achieve fitness goals including weight reduction, increased flexibility, youthful appearance, regulation of blood sugar and blood pressure levels, and popularly to promote peace within. Studies have proven the power of yoga to reverse brain aging as well.

The vast and diversified practice of yoga has been a compelling object of study for many researchers. Various studies prove beyond doubt the positive impact yoga has on health. One of the latest findings is the role yoga plays in reversing brain aging.

Aging of the brain has always been considered a natural occurrence, part and parcel of getting old. Memory loss, compromised flexibility, assisted living, and poor cognitive health later in life were all accepted as inevitable events. Yoga has proved otherwise, as is evident from the fact that regular yogic practitioners enjoy better quality of life than non-practitioners.

Scientists from Brazil formed two groups consisting of elderly women. One group consisted of women who had been practicing yoga for at least a few years. The other group consisted of healthy women who were not into yoga. The goal of the research was to analyze if the brain structure of yoga practitioners was different from that of non-practitioners. The scientists imaged the brains of women in both groups. Results proved that the prefrontal cortex of yoga practitioners was much thicker compared to that of non-practitioners. The prefrontal cortex is associated with memory and focus, which are generally lower as one advances in years. Thus, the study proved yoga's role in promoting cognitive strength and thereby preventing memory decline.

The structural changes that normally occur in an aging brain—including shrinkage—are minimized or prevented if yoga is practiced regularly. Those practicing yoga remain mentally alert in comparison to others of their age group. By supporting the structure and function of the brain, yoga effectively reverses brain aging. While starting young gives you optimum benefits, remember the rule that it is better late than never!

How Yoga Works For Brain

Some of the physical benefits of backbends, forward bends, stretches, lunges, twists, shoulder stands, handstands and headstands are easily recognized as you feel the stress, strain, pull and every other feeling associated with the physical part of the pose. If it is a backbend, you feel it in your hips, back, chest, shoulders and legs. You recognize instantly which parts are involved in the pose and the benefits of the particular practice. Yes, you are going to lose extra fat in your waist and abdomen, your back will get stronger and your flexibility will improve. Depending on the yoga pose, tension is felt in some areas more than the others. But what works for your brain is less obvious, as you do not feel it at the physical level. That is the way of yoga: It works even if you don't feel it. It works for your brain as much as it works for your body.

Various studies have proven that regular practice of yoga, meditation and pranayama keeps the brain young throughout the practitioner's life, thereby preventing age-related cognitive loss.

Here is how yoga works for brain:

Promotes Blood Flow

Proper flow of blood to the brain prevents memory lapses associated with aging. Blood flow to the brain decreases as one ages, and poor blood flow to the brain can result in stroke. Regular practice of yoga ensures your brain receives its share of oxygenated blood, thereby strengthening your cognitive skills, keeping your memory sound and reducing age-related health risks. Yoga inversions are a great way to boost the blood supply to your brain.

Increases Brain Volume and Improves Brain Chemistry

The cerebral cortex, which is associated with functions including thought and perception and is responsible for processing sensory information, thins as one ages. Regular practice of yoga and meditation thickens the cerebral cortex, thereby supporting optimum cognitive skills even as one gets older.

Gray matter loss is yet another change in the brain during aging. Loss of gray matter causes memory-related issues and cognitive loss. A reduced volume of gray matter is also a cause of age-related depression and emotional issues. By increasing gray matter volume, yoga supports cognitive function, emotional balance and keeps people free of depression as they get older.

Prevents Loss of Neurons in Brain

Neurons, the longest-lived cells in the body, can cause brain-related conditions when they die an unnatural death. Brain atrophy, a condition in which the brain loses neurons, affects the ability of cells to communicate. Alzheimer's and dementia can also cause brain atrophy.

Yoga poses, along with meditation practice, have been proven to be effective in reducing brain atrophy. Studies have also proven that yoga can be successful in slowing Alzheimer's progression. Regular yogic practice can also help prevent Alzheimer's.

Relieves Stress and Depression

Chronic stress can cause more damage than you might imagine. The hippocampus in the brain, which is responsible for memory, learning and emotions, is negatively affected by prolonged stress. Studies have proven that chronic stress in children and adolescents can result in behavioral issues. Adults who are chronically stressed develop poor cognitive function as they age. Stress-related damage to the prefrontal cortex and hippocampus affects memory power and understanding. For the aged, depression naturally follows. Depression also accelerates cellular aging, which again can be bad for the brain.

Regular practice of yoga is a great way to remain stress-free and with a balanced state of mind. Low levels of gamma-aminobutyric acid (GABA) are found in those who are stressed and depressed, but yoga increases GABA levels in the brain. Yoga poses, along with breathing techniques and meditation, improve GABA levels, relieve stress and promote calm.

Yoga works wonders regardless of when you start. Starting early helps to prevent health risks associated with aging; starting after the onset of a health condition can help cure the condition or at least assist in managing it and checking further progression. Either way, yoga helps—but isn't an ounce of prevention worth a pound of cure? While it's never too late to start practicing yoga, it's never too early either!

Yoga to Boost Brain Health

Yoga boosts immunity and thereby promotes overall health. However, practicing certain poses can specifically promote optimal brain health. Here is a list of important yoga poses to boost brain health.

Yoga Poses for Brain Health

Lotus Pose / Padmasana

Lotus pose is the best pose for meditation and an excellent pose to calm the brain. It increases awareness and boosts memory power. The pose soothes the nervous system and promotes peace.

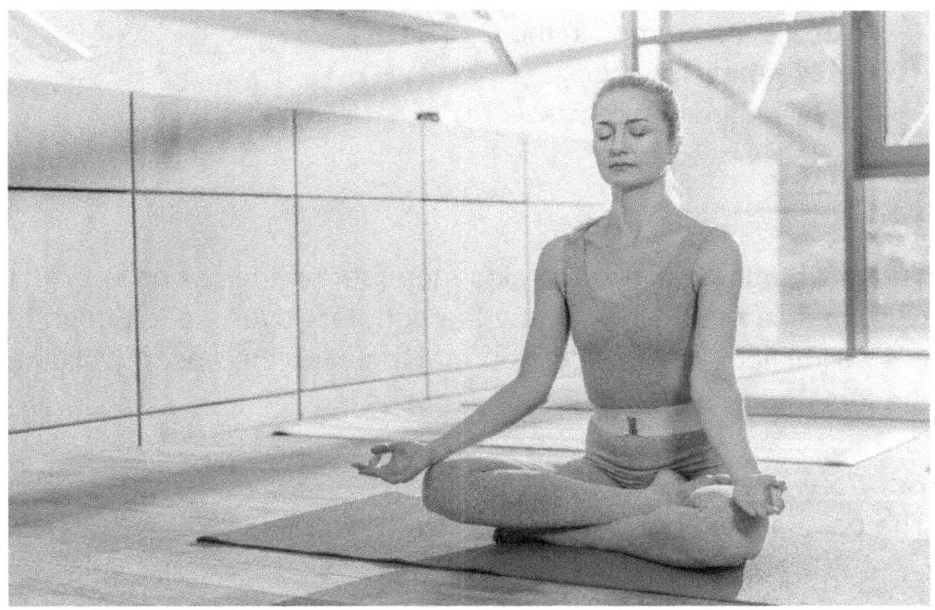

Instructions
1. Sit on the yoga mat with your spine straight. Keep your legs stretched in front of you.
2. Bend the right knee and place your right foot on the uppermost part of your left thigh. The right heel should touch the left side of your abdomen.
3. Bend your left knee over your right shin and place your left foot on the right thigh touching the abdomen.

4. Place your hands on your knees. Assume Chin Mudra, in which you bring the tips of your index finger and thumb together to form a circle. The other three fingers should be outstretched.
5. Close your eyes and your senses to the outside world.
6. Remain in the pose for one minute. With practice, the duration can be increased up to one hour.

Other Benefits

- Stretches the spine and tones your back
- Supports function of abdominal organs
- Relieves cramps in the legs
- Stretches the legs
- Strengthens the hips
- Relieves sciatica

Note

Those who find it difficult to place the feet on the opposite thighs can practice the pose with just the right foot over the left thigh. If it is still difficult to practice, you may practice the pose by sliding the feet under the thighs of the opposite legs.

Caution

The pose should not be practiced by those with:

- Severe knee injury
- Ankle injury

Thunderbolt Pose / Vajrasana

Thunderbolt Pose is another meditation pose. The pose may be challenging for those with lower flexibility levels in the legs. Being a meditation pose, it is effective in calming the mind and relieving stress. It is also effective in boosting concentration levels.

Thunderbolt Pose is the only yoga pose that can be performed after taking food.

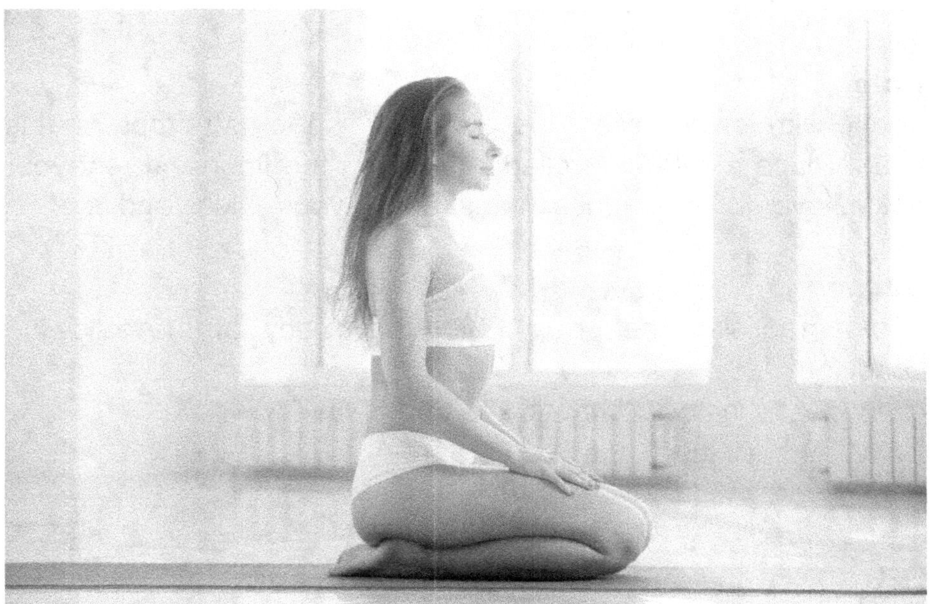

Instructions

1. Kneel down. The thighs should be close to each other.
2. Bring the big toes together while keeping your heels apart. Now your feet will resemble the letter 'V'.
3. Exhale as you lower your body.
4. Place your buttocks between your feet.
5. Keep your spine straight and your palms on your knees.

6. Remain in the pose for one minute. With practice, you can increase the duration to 20 to 30 minutes according to your comfort level.

Other Benefits

- Stretches the legs
- Improves blood flow to abdominal organs and promotes their function
- Improves digestion
- Relieves gas
- Relieves menstrual cramps

Note

Those with lower flexibility levels may wish to use props for this pose. Place a pillow or rolled blanket on the floor and rest your ankles over it. This reduces the stress to your ankles and legs.

Caution

Avoid practicing the pose if you have any of the following conditions:

- Knee injury or chronic knee problems
- Ankle injury

Reclining Thunderbolt Pose / Supta Vajrasana

Reclining Thunderbolt Pose can be more challenging than Thunderbolt Pose, as in this pose you lie on your back while your legs are still in Thunderbolt Pose. The pose promotes blood flow to the brain, which is essential for brain health. Regular practice of the pose relieves anxiety and depression.

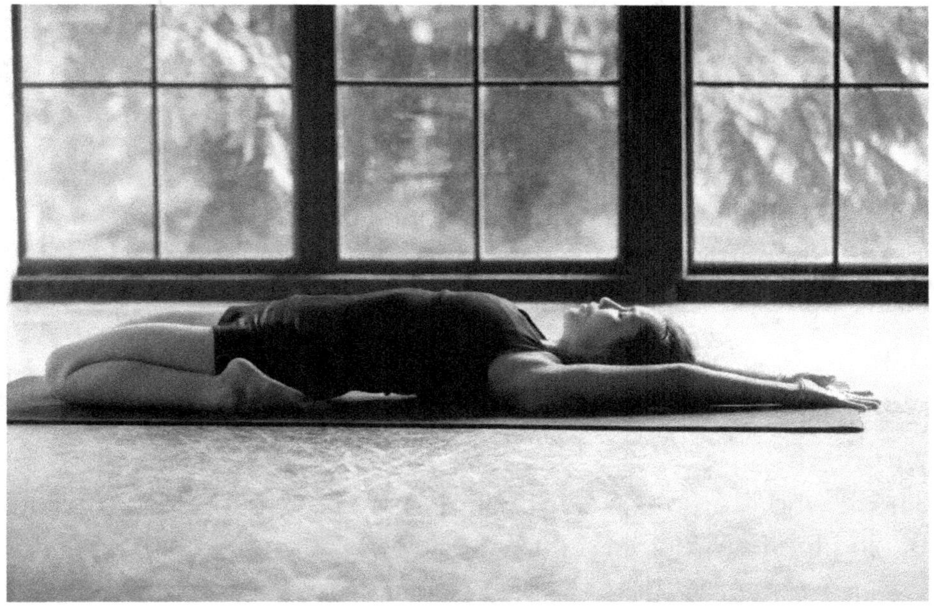

Instructions

1. Assume Thunderbolt Pose.
2. Hold your right foot with your right hand and your left foot with your left hand.
3. Place your right forearm on the ground while still holding your right foot.
4. Lower your left forearm to the floor. Now both your elbows will be on the ground with your body leaning backwards.

5. Release your elbows from the ground and gently lean further backwards and place your back on the floor.
6. Bring your arms over your shoulders. You can either keep your arms stretched upwards or hold the opposite shoulders with your forearms resting on the floor.
7. Remain in the pose for 30 seconds to one minute.
8. To get out of the pose, hold your feet, rest on your elbows, lift your back off the floor and come to Thunderbolt Pose. You may now release your legs and stretch them forward.

Other Benefits

- Strengthens the legs
- Stretches and tones the thighs
- Strengthens the back
- Stimulates function of abdominal organs
- Supports heart health
- Improves digestion
- Relieves constipation
- Boosts function of liver and kidneys

Note

Those who are unable to go all the way back can place a pillow behind the back and rest on the pillow.

Caution

Do not practice the pose if you have any of the following conditions:

- Headache
- Severe back injury
- Spinal issues
- Shoulder, hip or ankle injury
- Recent surgery
- Hernia

Half Lord of the Fishes Pose / Half-Spinal Twist / Ardha Matsyendrasana

Half Lord of the Fishes Pose is a twisted pose that strengthens and improves spine health. A healthy spine ensures brain health. Practicing this pose on a regular basis protects the brain from age-related disorders.

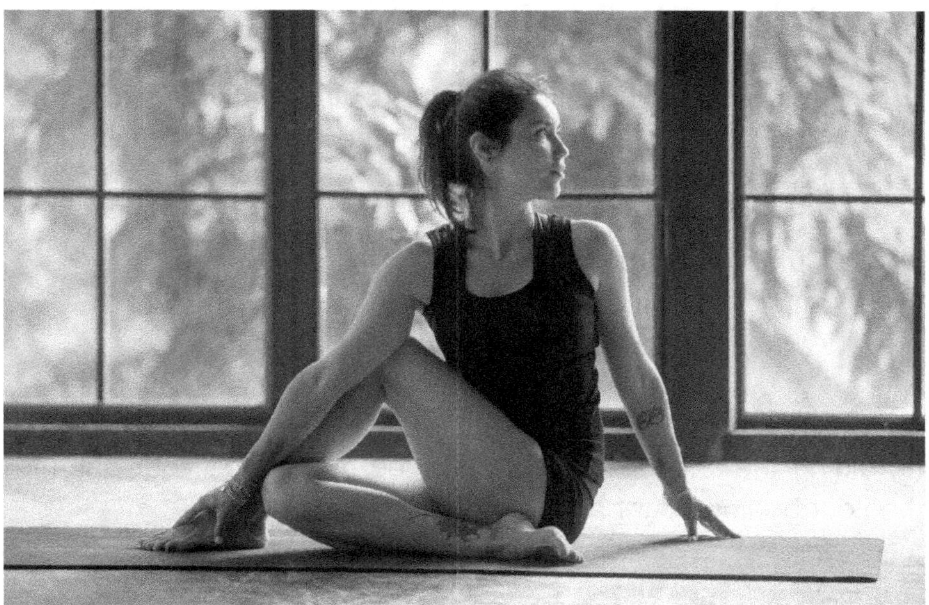

Instructions

1. Sit down with your legs stretched in front of you.
2. Draw your left leg towards you and over your right thigh to place the left foot on the outer side of the right hip.
3. Bend your right leg and place your right heel near your left buttock.
4. Turn the upper part of your body to your left.
5. Slide your left hand behind your back and hold the left ankle.

6. Lift your right hand upwards and bring it down over your left knee. Reach for your right knee and place the palm of your left hand on the right knee.
7. Turn your head towards your left. (Those with neck pain can look straight.)
8. Remain in the pose for one minute.
9. Release the pose and repeat on the other side.

Other Benefits
- Supports nervous system function
- Tones the back
- Improves lung health and relieves lung-related disorders
- Reduces excess fat in the abdomen and hips
- Strengthens liver and kidneys
- Cures tiredness
- Cures menstrual disorders
- Improves fertility
- Awakens kundalini power

Note
If holding the left ankle is difficult, you may place your palm on the floor behind your back.

Caution
The pose should not be practiced by those with:
- Back injury
- Spinal injury

Those with the following conditions should perform the pose with caution:
- Hyperthyroidism
- Hernia

Seated Forward Bend / Paschimotanasana

Seated Forward Bend increases blood flow to the brain, supports brain function, relieves stress and calms the mind. The pose stimulates and improves spine function, thereby supporting brain health.

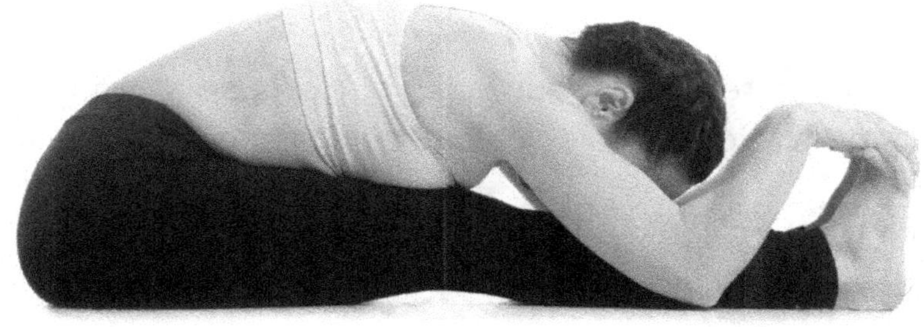

Instructions

1. Sit down and keep your legs stretched in front of you. Your toes should be pointed upwards and your spine straight.
2. Inhale while lifting your hands sideways and bring them over your head.
3. Exhale and bend forward, moving your hands along to hold the feet. Do not lift your knees.

4. Rest your forehead on the knees. If you can stretch further, you can place your forehead further down your legs.
5. Remain in the pose for 30 seconds.
6. Inhale as you slowly lift your torso and release your feet.

Other Benefits

- Stretches the back and tones back muscles
- Tones and improves function of abdominal organs
- Relieves digestive disorders
- Reduces belly fat
- Strengthens the nervous system
- Reduces excess fat in thighs and waist
- Cures menstrual disorders
- Stimulates kundalini power

Note

If it is difficult to reach for your feet, you can use a yoga strap to support your stretch, or hold your calves instead.

Caution

The pose should not be performed by those with the following conditions:

- Sciatic problems
- Slipped disc conditions

Sphinx Pose / Salamba Bhujangasana

A simple-to-perform backbend, Sphinx Pose tones your spine and promotes spine and brain health. It is a stress-reliever as well.

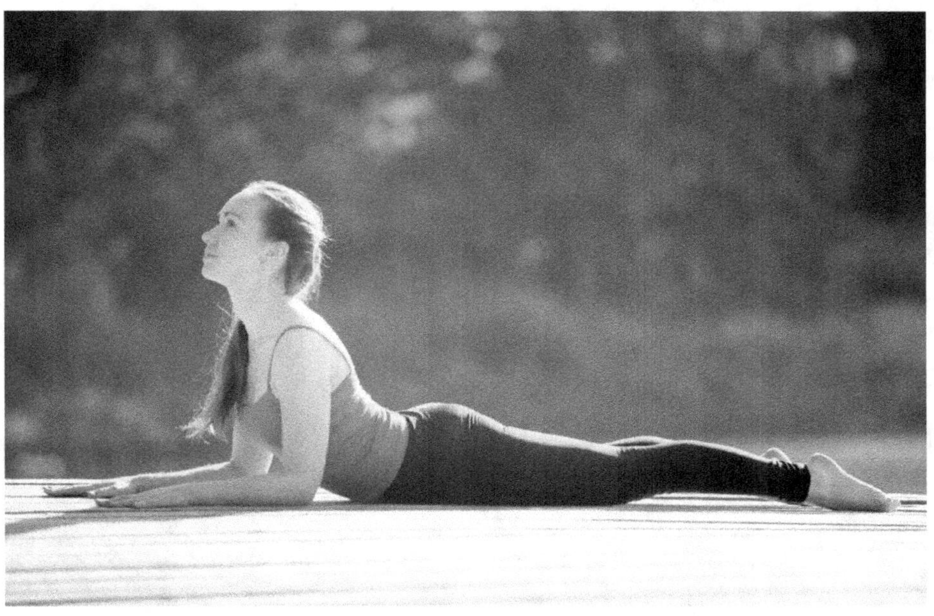

Instructions

1. Lie down on your stomach, keeping your feet together.
2. Stretch your arms forward and place your forearms on the floor, aligning your elbows under your shoulders.
3. With the forearms firmly pressed to the floor, inhale as you lift your head and chest off the ground. As you lift the upper part of your body as high as possible, your neck should be aligned to your spine.
4. Press your pubic bone firmly to the floor.
5. Contract your thighs and buttocks.
6. Keep your head straight.
7. Remain in the pose for 30 seconds to one minute.
8. Exhale as you slowly release the pose.

Other Benefits
- Expands the chest and improves lung function
- Stretches the shoulders
- Tones abdominal organs and improves their function
- Stimulates nervous system

Caution

The pose should not be practiced by those with the following conditions:
- Spine or back injury
- Recent abdominal surgery
- Pregnancy
- Severe injury in shoulders or arms

Cobra Pose / Bhujangasana

Cobra Pose is a backbend pose that supports spine flexibility and boosts spine and brain health. The pose promotes calm and is effective for curing mild depression.

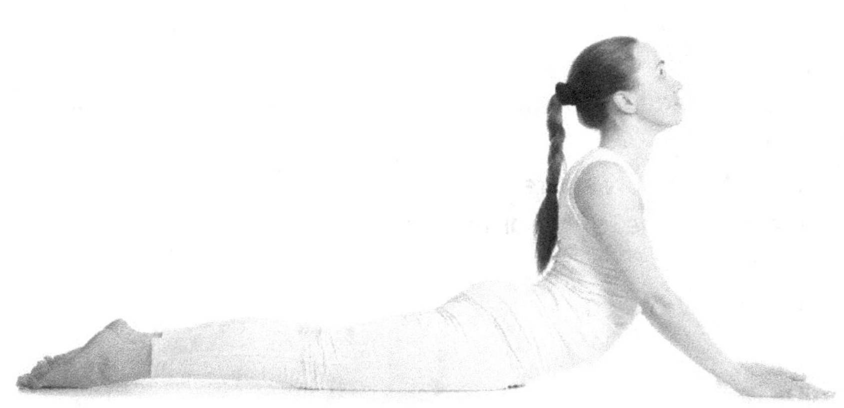

Instructions

1. Lie down on the floor on your stomach.
2. Place your palms by your chest with the elbows pointed upwards.
3. Inhale as you slowly lift your torso. Lift the upper part of your body till your hands are perpendicular to the ground.
4. Stretch your shoulders backwards and look straight.
5. Remain in the pose for 30 seconds.

Other Benefits

- Tones the back muscles
- Improves lung function and relieves respiratory disorders, including asthma

- Improves digestion
- Relieves neck pain
- Relieves menstrual cramps and other disorders associated with the menstrual cycle
- Helps to cure cervical spondylitis

Note

Those who are unable to lift their torso till their hands are straight can lift their head and chest initially. With practice, the pose can be mastered.

Caution

The pose should not be performed by those with the following health conditions:
- High blood pressure
- Carpal tunnel syndrome
- Hernia
- Hyperthyroidism

Bridge Pose / Setu Bandhasana

Yet another backbend pose, Bridge Pose is performed lying on the floor. The pose strengthens the spine, increases blood flow to the brain, and boosts brain function. It also promotes calm.

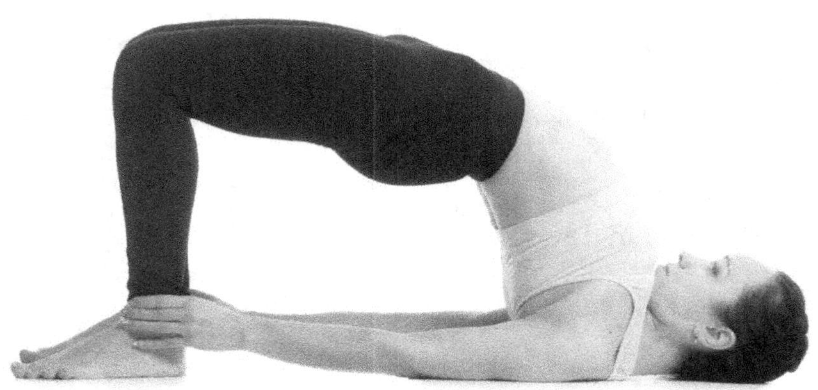

Instructions
1. Lie down on your back.
2. Place your feet hip-width apart on the floor by bending your legs. Your feet should be under your knees.
3. Place your hands at your sides with palms down.
4. Inhale while lifting your hips as high as possible. Your thighs should be parallel to each other.
5. Bring your hands together and clasp them together on the floor. Alternatively, you can place your hands by the sides.
6. Remain in the pose for 30 seconds.
7. Exhale as you slowly place your back on the floor.

Other Benefits
- Expands the chest and improves lung function
- Tones the back
- Supports thyroid function
- Strengthens the digestive system
- Lowers high blood pressure
- Cures symptoms associated with menopause

Note
If lifting the hips high is difficult, you may place a block under your hips.

Caution
The pose should not be practiced by those with the following conditions:
- Neck injury
- Shoulder injury

Shoulder Stand / Sarvangasana

Called the Queen of Yoga Poses, Shoulder Stand is one of the best poses to increase blood flow to the brain. The pose promotes calm.

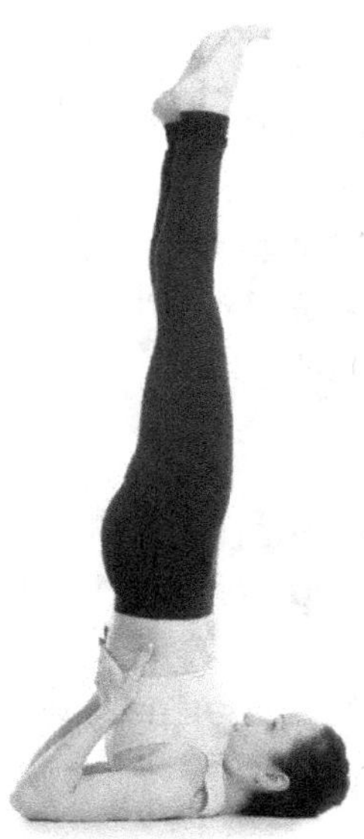

Instructions

1. Lie down on your back with your hands by your sides.
2. Exhale as you lift your legs, hips and back so the body is perpendicular to your neck. Keep your knees straight.
3. Bend your hands and place your palms behind your back to support your body.
4. Keep your eyes closed. Alternatively, you can look at your toes.
5. Remain in the pose for one minute.
6. Release the pose by lowering your legs towards your head before releasing your hands from your back.
7. Slowly place your back and legs on the floor.

Other Benefits
- Boosts immune power
- Energizes the whole body
- Improves lung function and relieves respiratory disorders, including asthma
- Stimulates glands and promotes their function
- Effective for thyroid disorders
- Aids in detoxification
- Maintains youthfulness
- Improves function of reproductive organs
- Prevents headache
- Improves varicose veins
- Maintains blood sugar levels
- Maintains healthy weight

Note
If performing Shoulder Stand is difficult, you may use wall support by placing your legs on the wall.

If you are practicing with a partner, you may have your partner hold your legs.

Caution
The pose is not recommended for conditions including:
- High blood pressure
- Pregnancy
- Menstruation
- Heart ailments
- Brain disease
- Severe eye problems
- Slipped disc
- Cervical spondylitis
- Severe back or spine problems
- Shoulder, arm or neck injury

While the pose is effective in preventing headaches, it should not be performed while one is experiencing a headache.

Plough Pose / Halasana

Plough Pose promotes blood flow to the brain and supports brain health. Practicing the pose helps to calm the mind.

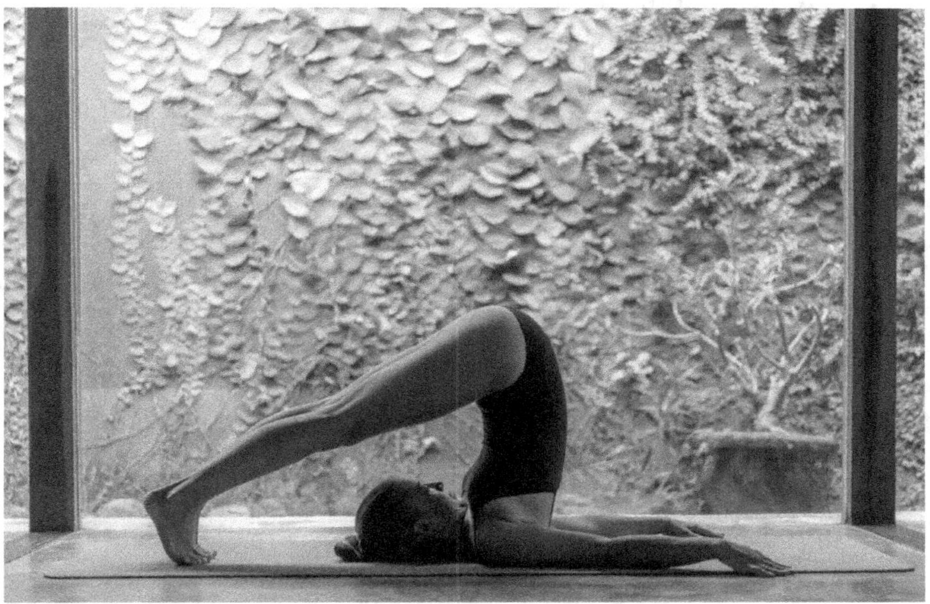

Instructions

1. Lie down on your back with your hands by your sides.
2. Exhale as you lift your legs up and towards your head.
3. Lower your legs and place your toes on the floor behind your head. If you find it difficult to lift your hips upwards, you can support your back by pressing your palms against it.
4. Stretch your legs as far as possible from your head so your chin and chest are in contact.
5. Keep your hands stretched on the floor.
6. Remain in the pose for one minute.

Other Benefits
- Boosts immunity
- Postpones symptoms of aging
- Supports function of thyroid glands
- Improves lung function and relieves respiratory disorders
- Reduces tummy fat
- Stretches the spine
- Strengthens the nerves
- Tones the back and relieves back pain, particularly lower back pain
- Stimulates abdominal organs and improves their function
- Cures insomnia

Note
If placing the legs on the floor behind your head is difficult, place them on a block. As your flexibility improves, you will be able to lower your legs to the floor.

Caution
Those with the following conditions should refrain from practicing the pose:
- Neck injury
- Shoulder injury
- Back or spinal injury
- High blood pressure
- Diarrhea

Headstand / Sirsasana

Headstand, rightly called the King of Poses, is a challenging yoga pose with wonderful benefits. In this pose, you stand on your head, which causes your brain to receive increased blood flow that provides nourishment to brain cells. Practicing Headstand improves brain health and boosts memory power and focus. The pose promotes a sense of balance and calm.

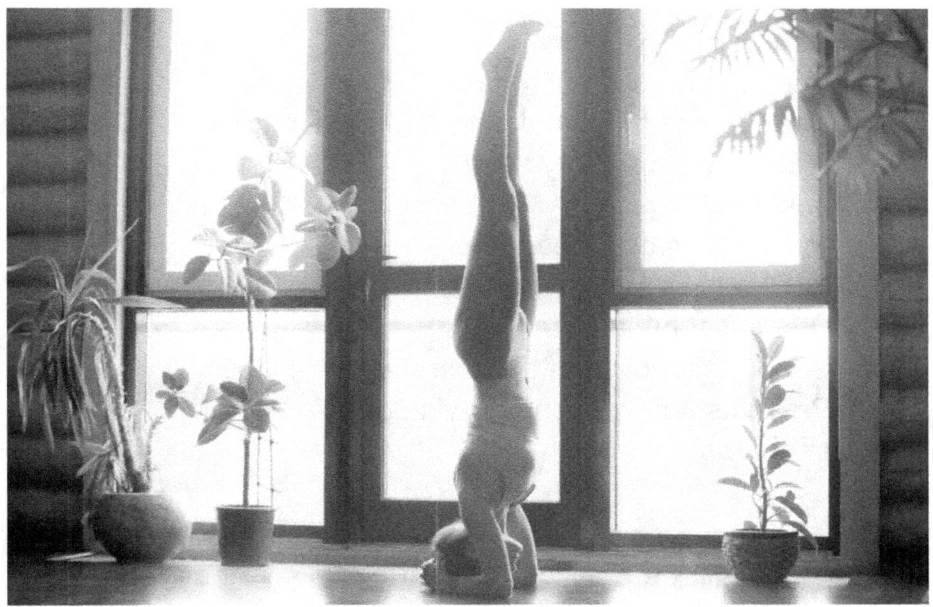

Instructions

1. Go down on your knees.
2. Place your forearms on the floor. Interlock your fingers to form a cup-like shape with your palms.
3. Place the crown of your head on the palms.
4. Lift your knees off the floor, raising your hips to support the lift.
5. Walk your feet towards your head. Get as close as possible, so your hips are over your shoulders.

6. Focusing on your body's alignment and balance, lift your legs slowly off the floor towards the ceiling.
7. Once you are confident you are balanced, straighten your legs so you are in a straight line from head to feet.
8. Keep your eyes closed.
9. Remain in the pose for a few seconds initially. With practice, you can increase the duration up to 5 minutes. However, yoga texts suggest that you can remain in the pose as long as you can comfortably hold it.

Other Benefits

- Supports function of the endocrine glands
- Strengthens the shoulders, arms and back
- Improves respiratory function
- Improves digestion
- Relieves chronic headache
- Relieves menstrual disorders
- Cures insomnia
- Supports function of the reproductive glands
- Prevents hair loss and graying of hair
- Improves vision

Note

The pose should be practiced after performing other yoga poses and before breathing techniques and meditation.

Beginners should practice the pose only under able guidance. Those who find it difficult to balance in this pose can practice the pose close to a wall so the legs can be supported.

Caution

The pose should not be practiced if the practitioner has any of the following health conditions:

- Spondylitis
- Slipped disc
- High blood pressure
- Heart disease
- Severe glaucoma
- Brain hemorrhage
- Menstruation
- Pregnancy
- Kidney problems

Breathing Techniques for Brain Health

Pranayama, the breathing techniques, are an inevitable part of yoga practice. Regular practice of breathing techniques has amazing health benefits to offer. Breathing techniques are generally considered to be effective for calming the mind and aiding in spiritual elevation. The fact is that they have even more to offer. These techniques not only balance the mind but also promote physical health and brain health.

Some of the important breathing techniques to boost brain health include:

Alternate Nostril Breathing / Nadi Shodhana

Alternate Nostril Breathing calms the mind. It improves focus and prepares the body and mind for effective meditation.

Instructions

1. Choose a calm place with fresh air.
2. Sit in Lotus Pose or Easy Pose. Your spine should be straight.
3. Perform Chin Mudra with your left hand by bringing the tips of the thumb and index finger together in slight contact. The remaining fingers should be outstretched.
4. Fold the index and middle fingers of your right hand so the fingers touch the base of the right thumb.
5. Close the right nostril with your right thumb as the ring and little fingers remain stretched.

6. Inhale through your left nostril deeply into your belly. Mentally observe your breath as it travels down your stomach.
7. Close the left nostril with the ring and little fingers of your right hand. As you close the left, release your right nostril and exhale slowly through your right nostril.
8. After exhaling fully, inhale through the right nostril with the left nostril still closed.
9. Now close your right nostril with your thumb and release the left nostril and exhale slowly. This is the completion of one round of Alternate Nostril Breathing.
10. Perform 5 to 10 rounds.
11. On completing the breathing technique, place your hands on your knees and take a few normal breaths.

Other Benefits

- Improves oxygen flow
- Purifies all energy channels
- Increases circulation
- Strengthens the nervous system
- Improves respiratory function
- Detoxifies the body
- Balances the right and left hemispheres of the brain

Note

Practice Alternate Nostril Breathing only on an empty stomach. The technique is best performed early in the morning.

Exhalation of breath should take longer than inhalation.

Humming Bee Breath / Bhramari Breathing

Humming Bee Breath relieves stress and calms the mind. The practice improves memory and focus.

Instructions

1. Choose a place where you can sit quietly while enjoying some fresh air.
2. Sit in Lotus Pose or Thunderbolt Pose. You may also sit in Easy Pose. You should be comfortable in the pose so you can focus on breathing.
3. Keep your back straight and the body relaxed. Keep your eyes closed.
4. Observe the feeling of quietness in you.
5. Keep your lips closed and your teeth slightly apart. Place the tip of your tongue on the space behind your front upper teeth. Keep your jaw relaxed.
6. Bend your hands and bring the palms towards your face.
7. Close the ears with your thumbs by gently pressing against the cartilage.
8. Place your index fingers on your forehead above the eyebrows.
9. Bring your middle finger, ring finger and little finger over your eyes to touch the bridge of the nose with the tips of these fingers.
10. Focus on the area between your eyebrows.
11. Inhale deeply through your nostrils so your belly expands with the breath.
12. Lock your chin with your chest.
13. Exhale slowly, releasing a low-pitched humming sound (something like 'hmmmm') from the back of your throat. This sound is similar to the sound of bees humming, hence the name for this breathing technique.

14. Straighten your neck as you exhale.
15. Remember to keep the tip of your tongue in the same position as mentioned above.
16. Feel the vibration throughout your body, from the crown of your head till your toes.
17. Do four repetitions. Inhalation and exhalation can be as long as you are comfortable with.
18. Breathe quietly a few times after you complete Bhramari.
19. Once you have completed the practice, mentally observe yourself before you slowly open your eyes.

Other Benefits

- Boosts function of pineal and pituitary glands
- Regulates blood pressure
- Promotes sleep
- Improves voice quality
- Relieves anger
- Cures headache
- Boosts self-confidence

Note

Just like all the yoga poses except Thunderbolt Pose, breathing techniques should be practiced on an empty stomach. Ideal times for practicing Bhramari are early morning and late night.

Caution

Bhramari is best avoided by those with the following conditions:

- Ear infection
- Heart pain
- Epilepsy
- Very high blood pressure

Meditation

Meditation is one of the best ways to maintain brain health. Meditation calms the mind, relieves stress and promotes peace. It promotes a positive mental attitude and boosts your self-confidence. It increases self-awareness as well. Regular practice of meditation strengthens immunity. Meditation promotes mental clarity and creativity. It's amazingly effective for managing or relieving anger.

How to Meditate

Instructions

- Everyone has a purpose to achieve through meditation. It can be to promote peace within, improve concentration, promote health, or manage anger, fear, stress or depression—in short, anything that one does not already possess. Identify your purpose and define it before you set out to meditate.
- If you intend to do mantra meditation, choose an appropriate mantra.
- Choose a calm place that is properly ventilated.
- Now that you are ready with the basics, get into action by sitting in any meditation pose. You can perform Lotus Pose, Thunderbolt Pose, Easy Pose or Accomplished Pose.
- Inhale and exhale slowly.
- Focus your mind on your breath.
- If you have an affirmation, this is the time to focus on your affirmation.

- From here, there are absolutely no hard and fast rules. You can visualize your affirmation or you can focus on your breath. You can chant a mantra or mentally observe the inner you.
- Sit in meditation as long as you can remain focused.

Note

Though incense is used in some yoga studios while practicing yoga and meditation, it is generally recommended not to use incense during your practice. Apart from the fact that it causes respiratory issues in some people, it can also distract you from your practice. Essential oils, though, are recommended. Extracts of herbs, trees and various plant materials, they are natural products that have a calming effect. Using essential oils that calm the mind is optional, but you may find that it is the right choice while you practice meditation.

Super Brain Yoga

The name sounds compelling, but the earlier pages of this book have already listed yoga poses that boost brain health. What, then, is Super Brain Yoga? As the name suggests, this is an excellent practice to promote brain health. It is also a routine practice in the land of yoga, albeit for religious reasons. The ancients of every land gained supremacy over their bodies, minds and souls in their own ways, but as their knowledge travelled down through the generations, things took a different form—at least in the land of yoga, where every practice was associated with religion.

A fully developed human brain has 300 million neurons connecting the right side to the left. The way the brain functions is amazing beyond words, but old age can steal some or most of that function if the brain is not exercised as one would exercise the body.

How Super Brain Yoga Works

Super Brain Yoga has been proven very effective in improving brain function. Research conducted by Dr. Joie P. Jones from the Department of Radiological Sciences at the University of California proves the effectiveness of Super Brain Yoga. The study proves that the energy centers, which are acupuncture points, are activated in this practice. The ear lobe holds acupressure points for various organs, including the brain. Practicing this exercise activates all energy centers and boosts brain health.

How to Do Super Brain Yoga

Instructions

- Stand facing the east.
- Touch the roof of your mouth with your tongue. This should be maintained throughout the practice.
- Bend your left hand and hold the right earlobe with your thumb and index finger. Your thumb should hold the front part of the earlobe and your index finger the back. Your left forearm should be close to your chest.
- With your right hand thumb and index finger, hold your left earlobe the same way as you are holding the right. Your right forearm should cross over your left.
- Pressing both ears, inhale slowly as you lower your body towards the ground. Your heels should remain in place as you squat.
- Remain in the position for 2 seconds.
- Exhale as you get back to a standing position, still holding your ears.
- Repeat this exercise 10 times. With practice you can perform this exercise for about 10 minutes.

Benefits

- Synchronizes the right and left brain hemispheres
- Energizes the brain
- Stimulates brain function
- Boosts memory power
- Increases mental alertness
- Boosts creative skills
- Improves mental clarity
- Relieves stress
- Promotes peace

Note

Super Brain yoga can be performed both in the morning and evening on an empty stomach.

Caution

The exercise should not be performed during menstruation. Those who have sleep problems should perform Super Brain yoga only in the morning.

Conclusion

I hope that you enjoyed reading the book and found it to be rich in information which you can put to use immediately and in years to come.

We have carefully worded the instructions so they can be clearly understood even by those who are new to yoga. We hope the images we have chosen to accompany the instructions help you with your practice as well.

We highly recommend that you keep practicing the poses mentioned in the book for about 3 months to track your progress. A pose that seems tough on Day 1 should be easily accomplished in a few weeks. Since all the poses support brain health, we are sure they will help you to achieve your goals, even ones that seem far-fetched now.

Also by Noah Miller

You might also enjoy my other yoga books:

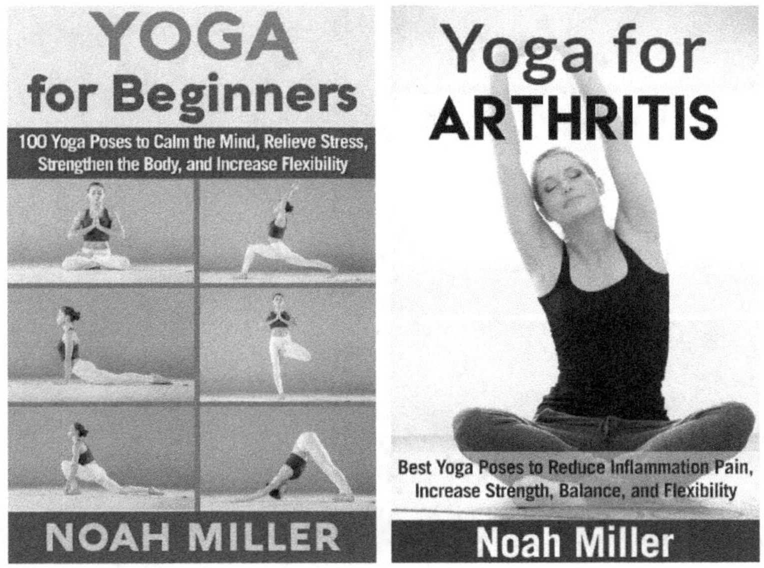